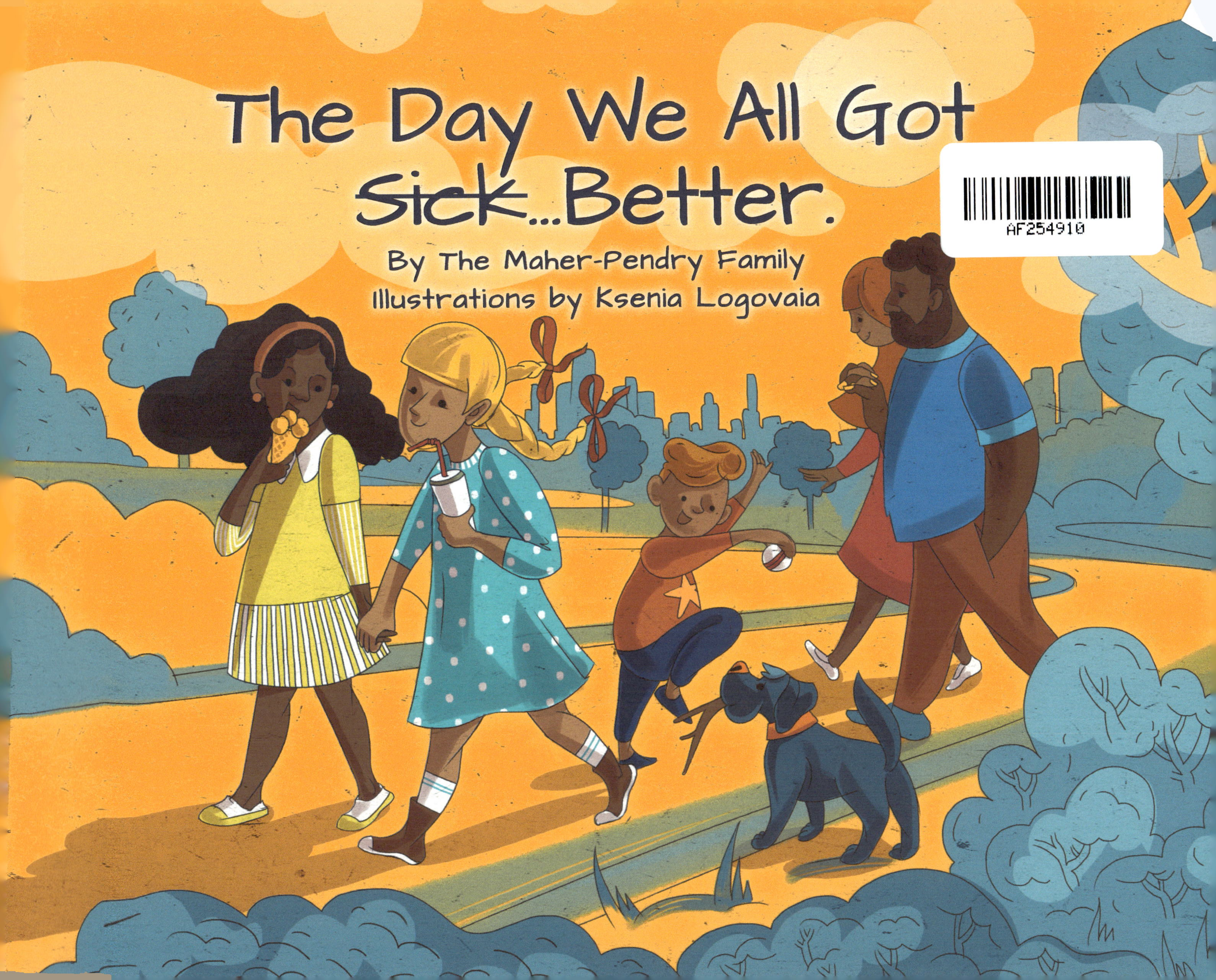

The Day We All Got Sick...Better.
By The Maher-Pendry Family
Illustrations by Ksenia Logovaia
AF254910

The Day We All Got Sick Better

Printed in the United States of America

Hardcover ISBN: 978-1-960876-57-7
Paperback ISBN: 978-1-960876-58-4
Ebook ISBN: 978-1-960876-59-1

Library of Congress Control Number: 2023923023

Muse Literary
3319 N. Cicero Avenue
Chicago IL 60641-9998

For:

A teacher named Amy Przygoda, who cared
for us beyond the classroom

and

A nurse named Kelly Trainor, who taught us
how to move forward beyond recovery.

Without all you did, there could be no us as
we are today: healed and whole.
We are forever grateful.

Advance Praise

"The Maher-Pendry family shares colorful page after page of images and emotional snapshots - the inner thoughts of the just-right "First Aid" for young families wrestling with the competing needs of all when illness or injury enters the home. As readers we learn, feel, and receive comfort from the carefully chosen words on each page.
The Maher-Pendry family's account of how lives are called to change to support Sister's healing process reminds readers that supporting the healing of one through the eyes and efforts of many is essential and life-changing."
-Jacqueline Griesdorn, M.ed., Ph.D., MS Child Development / Bilingual Education Specialization

"As a Certified Child Life Specialist, the impact an illness has on the entire family system is crucial to understanding how to best support our pediatric patients. The Day We All Got Sick…Better, captures the complex and nuanced effects of illness, allowing patients and families encountering similar experiences to feel heard, understood and not alone. I highly recommend this book to children going through medical experiences, as well as their siblings, for better comprehension and a sense of commonality."
-Nicole Brosnan, MS, CCLS

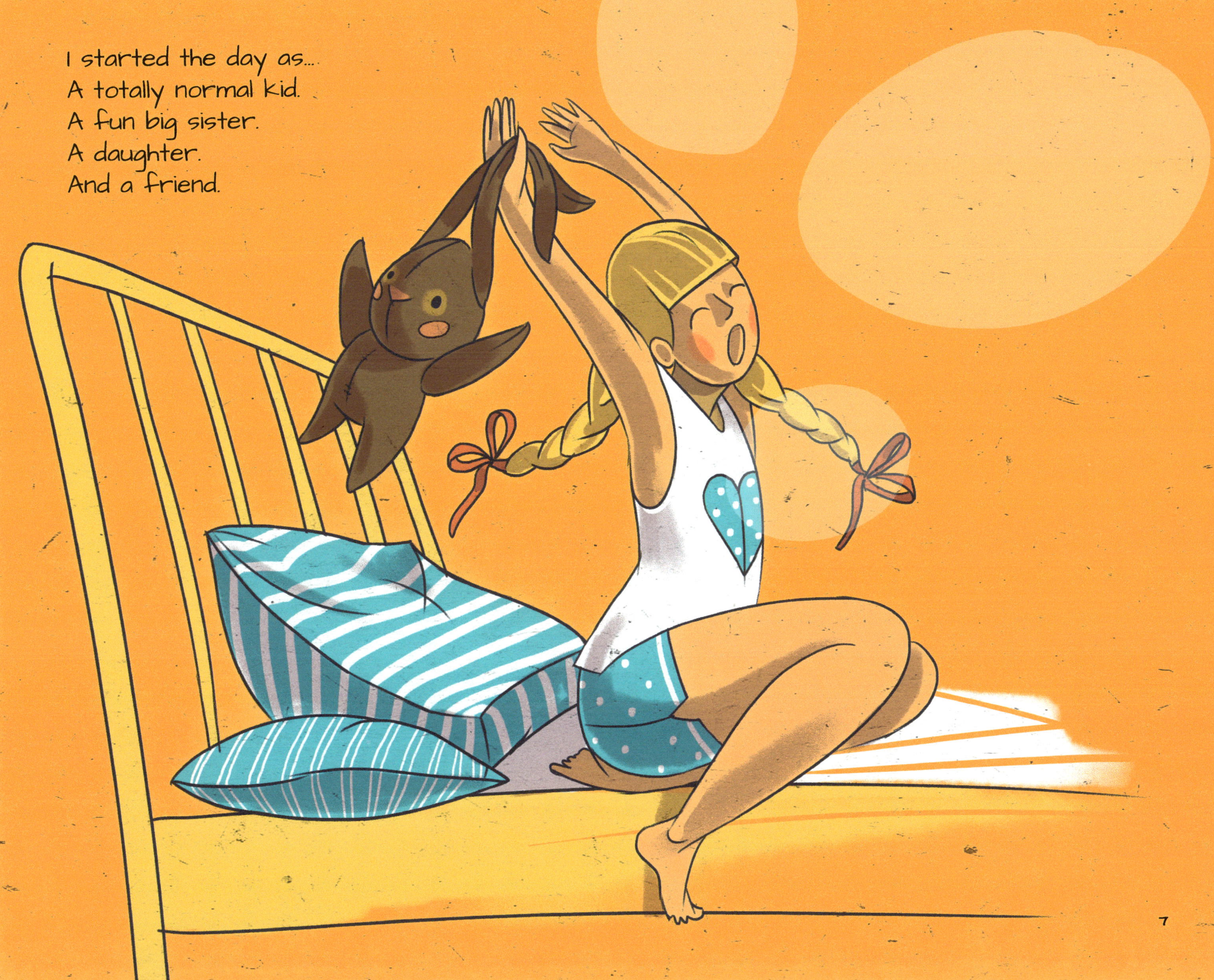

I started the day as....
A totally normal kid.
A fun big sister.
A daughter.
And a friend.

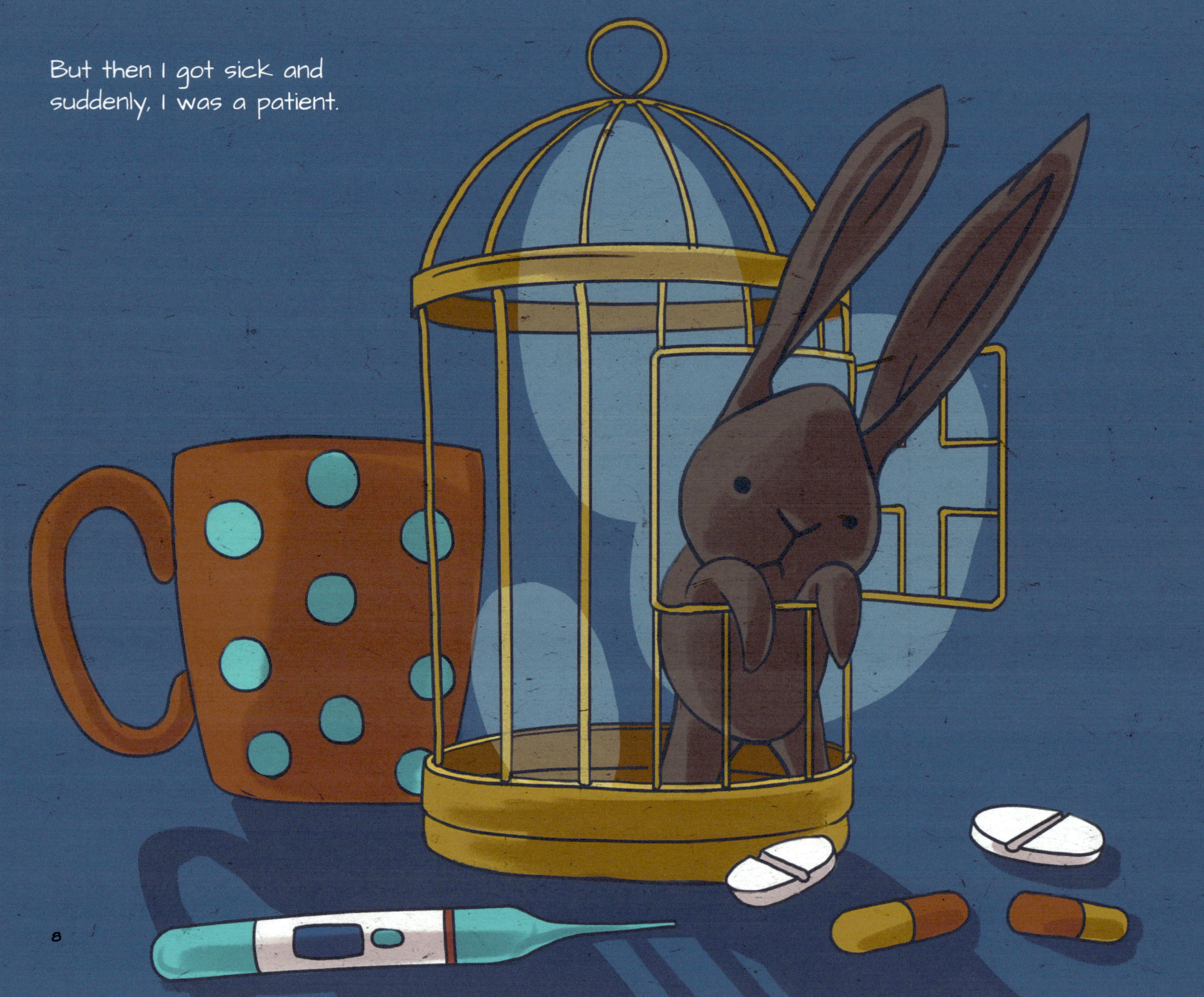

8

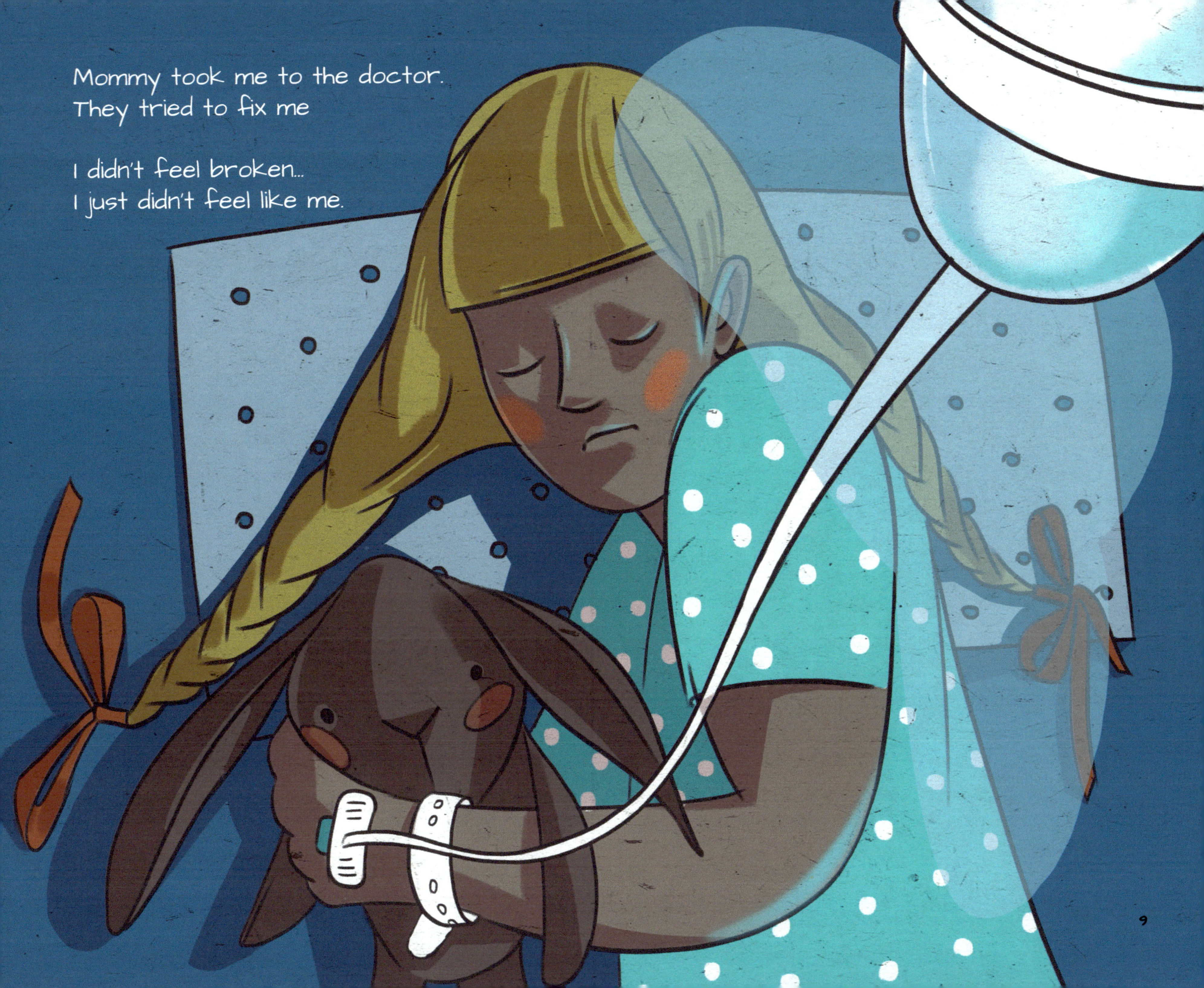

Mommy took me to the doctor.
They tried to fix me

I didn't feel broken...
I just didn't feel like me.

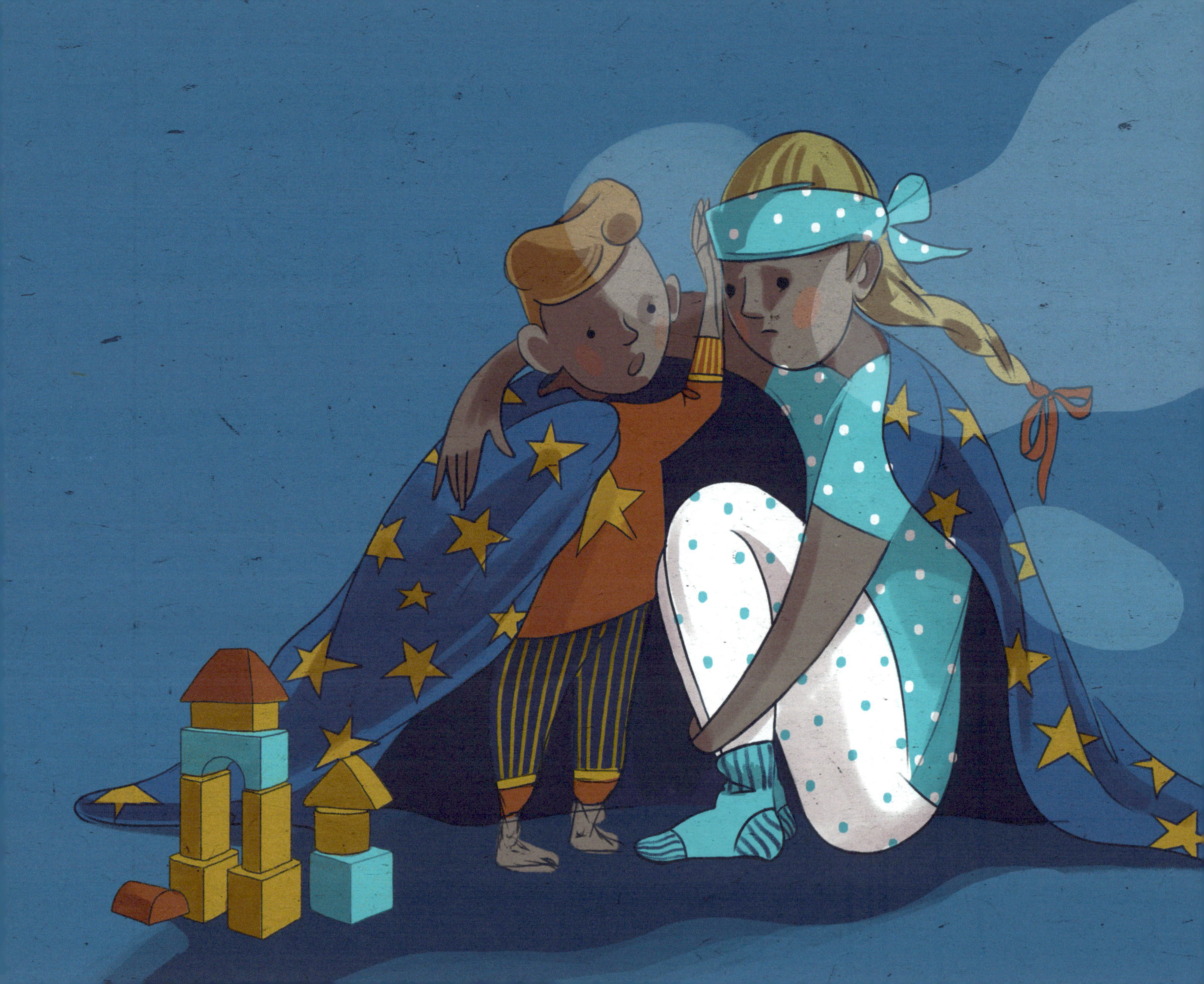

When my big sister got sick,
I didn't know what to do.

I'm just a little brother.

I asked over and over if she
was okay. She didn't say much.

She was sad and so was I.

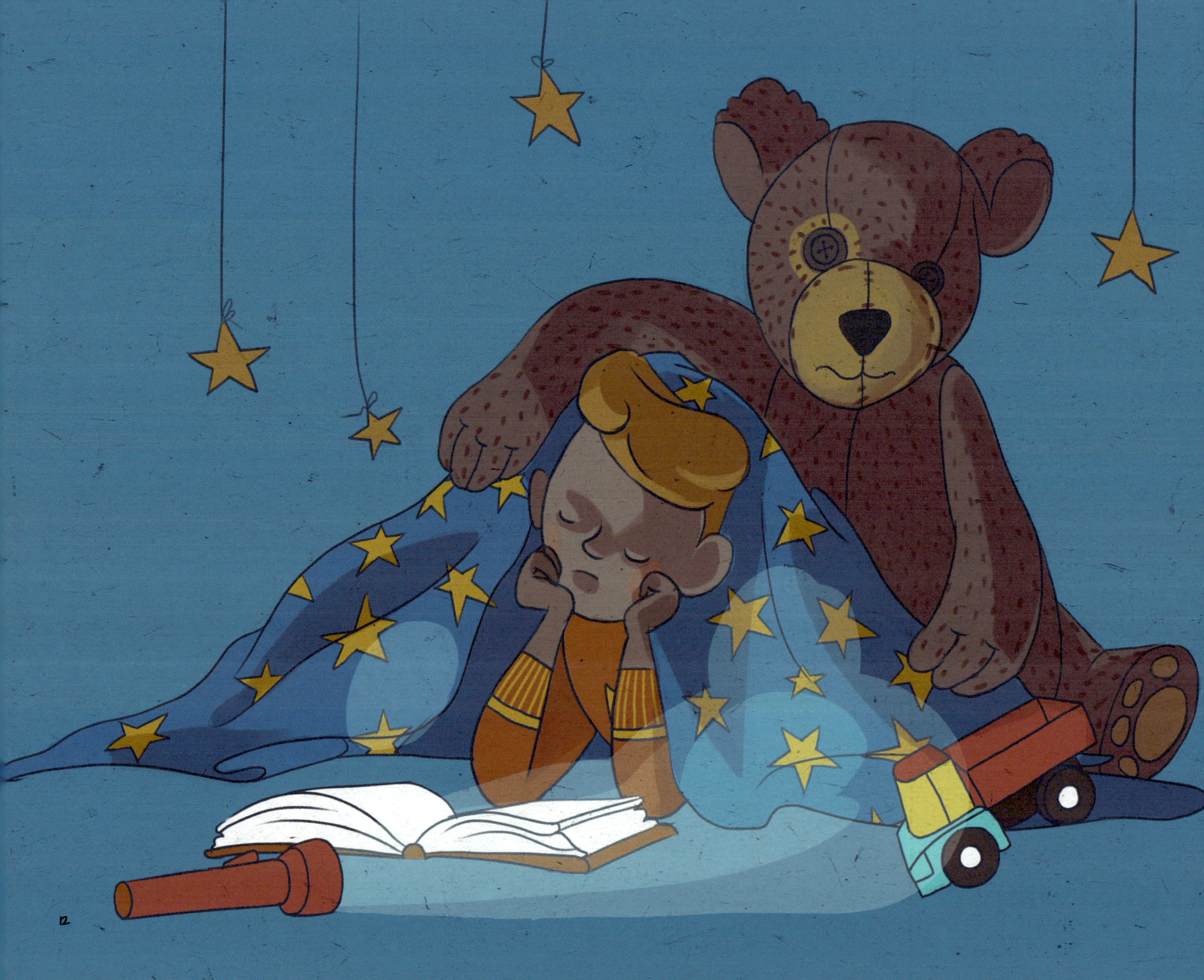

12

When my big sister got sick,
she was hardly ever home.

She was always with doctors
or with Mommy.

I really missed her... and Mommy.

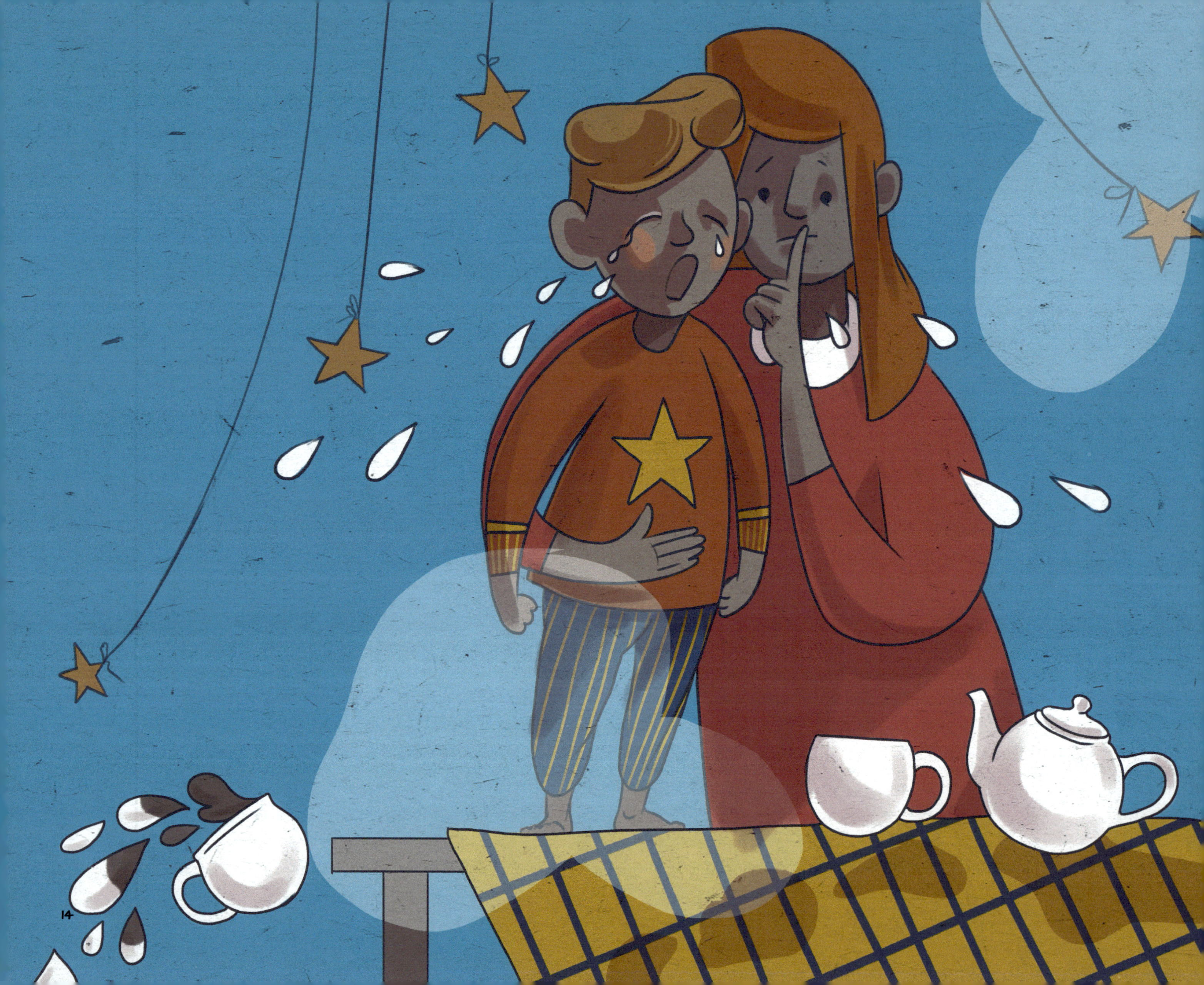

When she was home I wasn't
allowed to jump around, make a
lot of noise, or watch any of my
shows.

Sometimes it felt like everyone was
mad at me.

I kind of got sick of it.

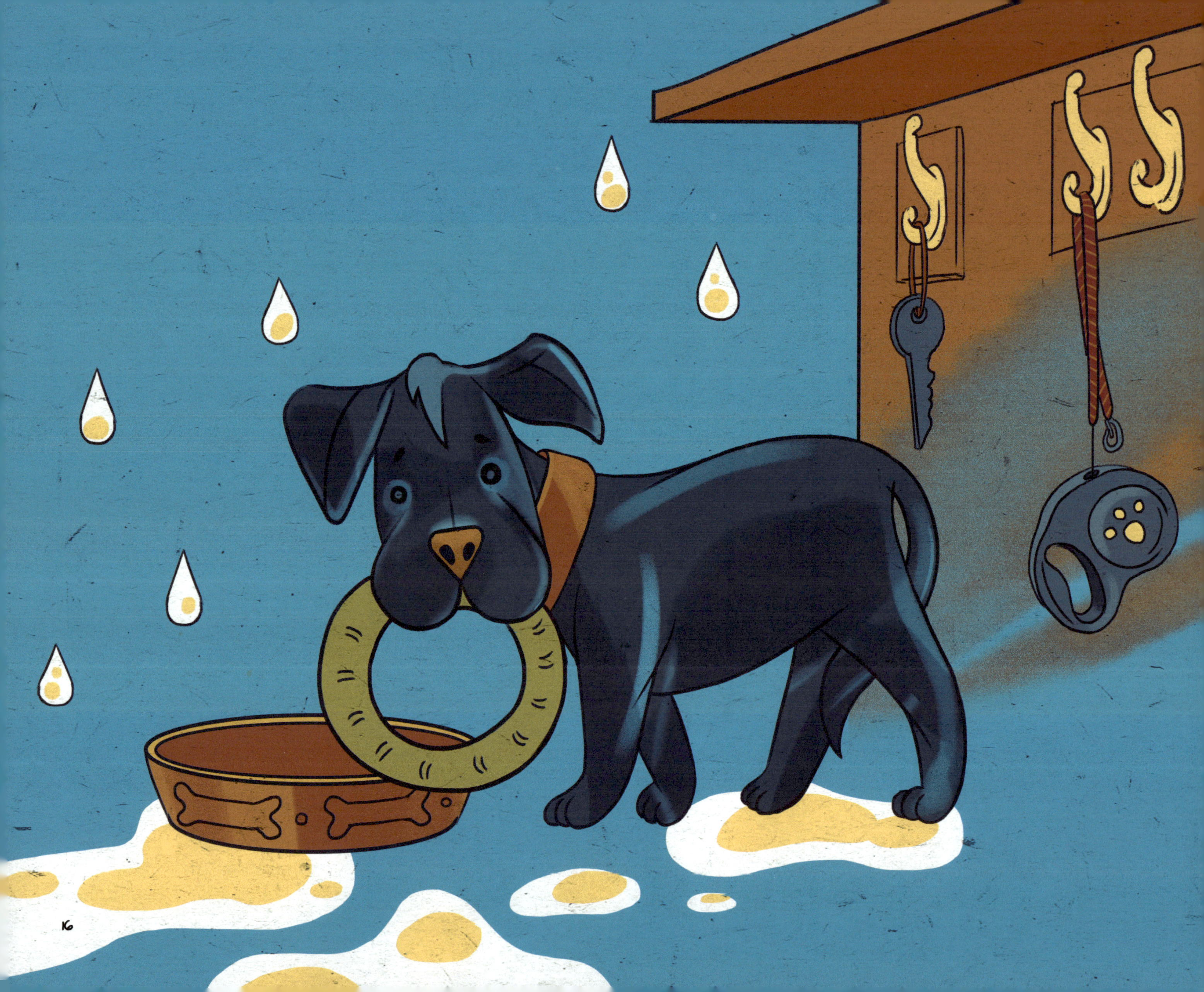

When the big girl got sick, the house
was empty and quiet.

Even when it was full of humans, it
was quiet.

I didn't get to play as much.
I didn't go for walks that much.
And sometimes that was a problem...
Because I REALLLLY had to go
potty.

And I also got REALLLLY bored.

I would go looking for fun things to do.
Only, everyone else called it "looking for trouble."

I chewed and ate everything and anything
I could (which was a fun thing to do!)

But then both the big girl and I were sick!
(Mine was a lot messier...and definitely not fun.)

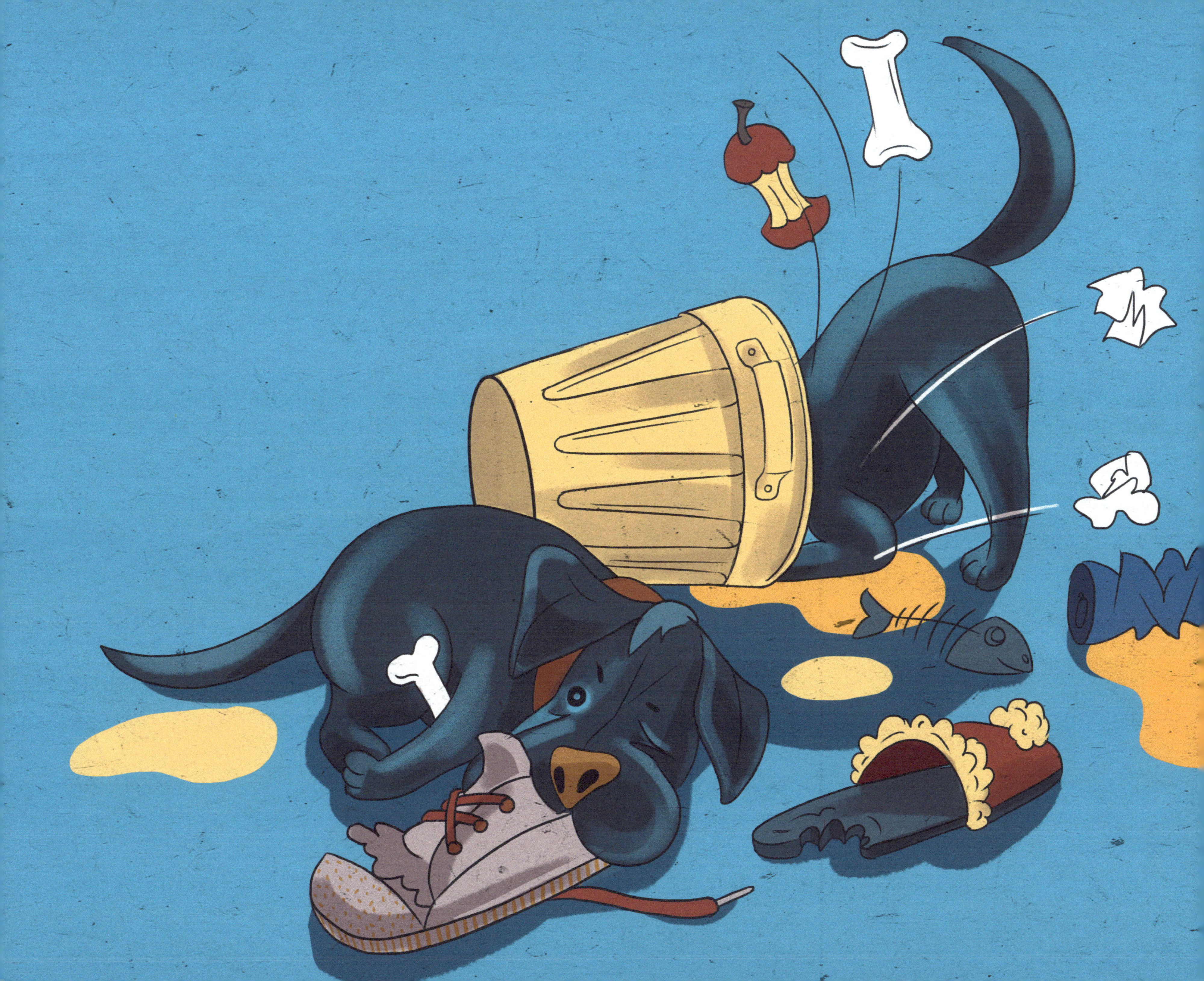

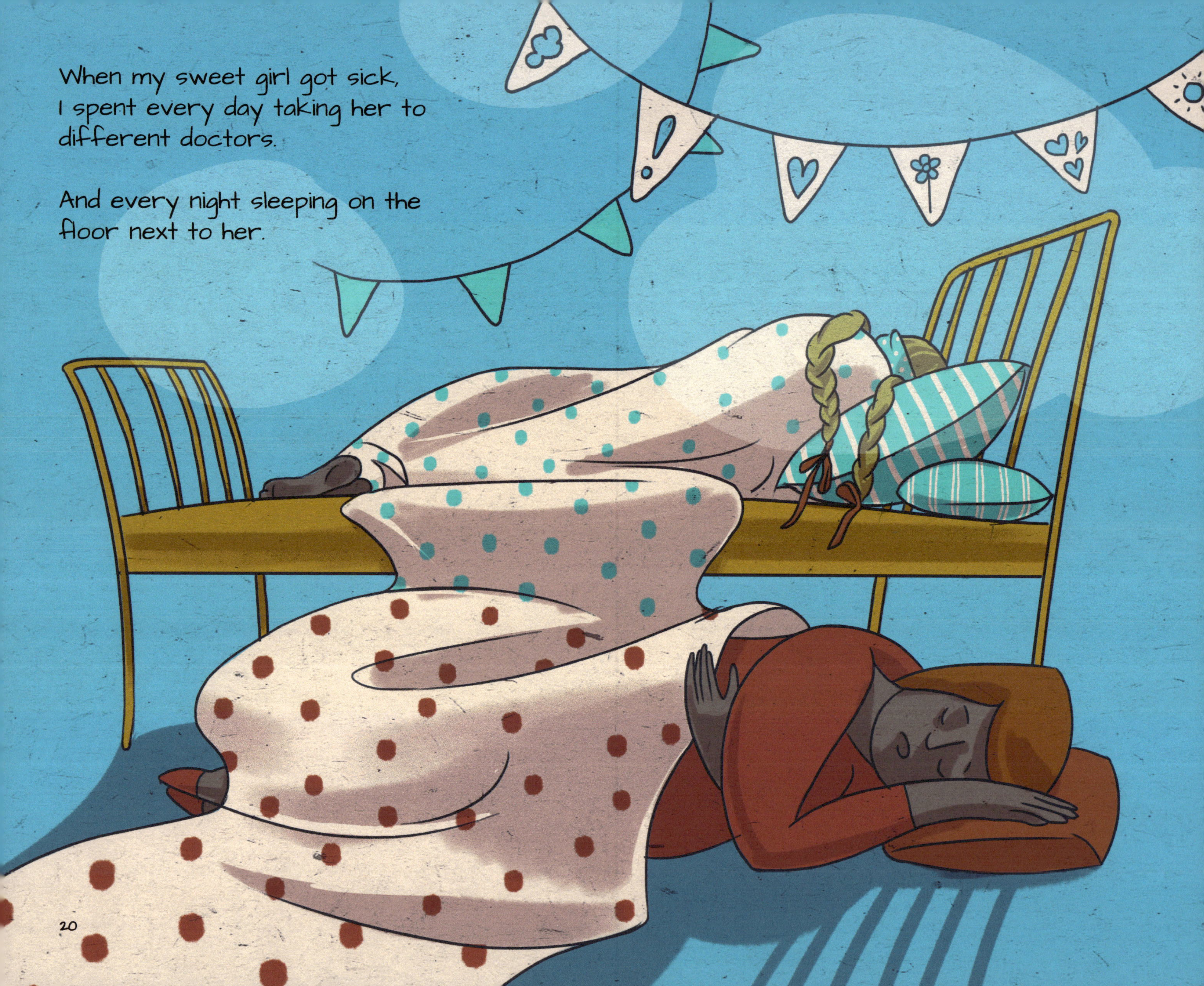

When my sweet girl got sick,
I spent every day taking her to
different doctors.

And every night sleeping on the
floor next to her.

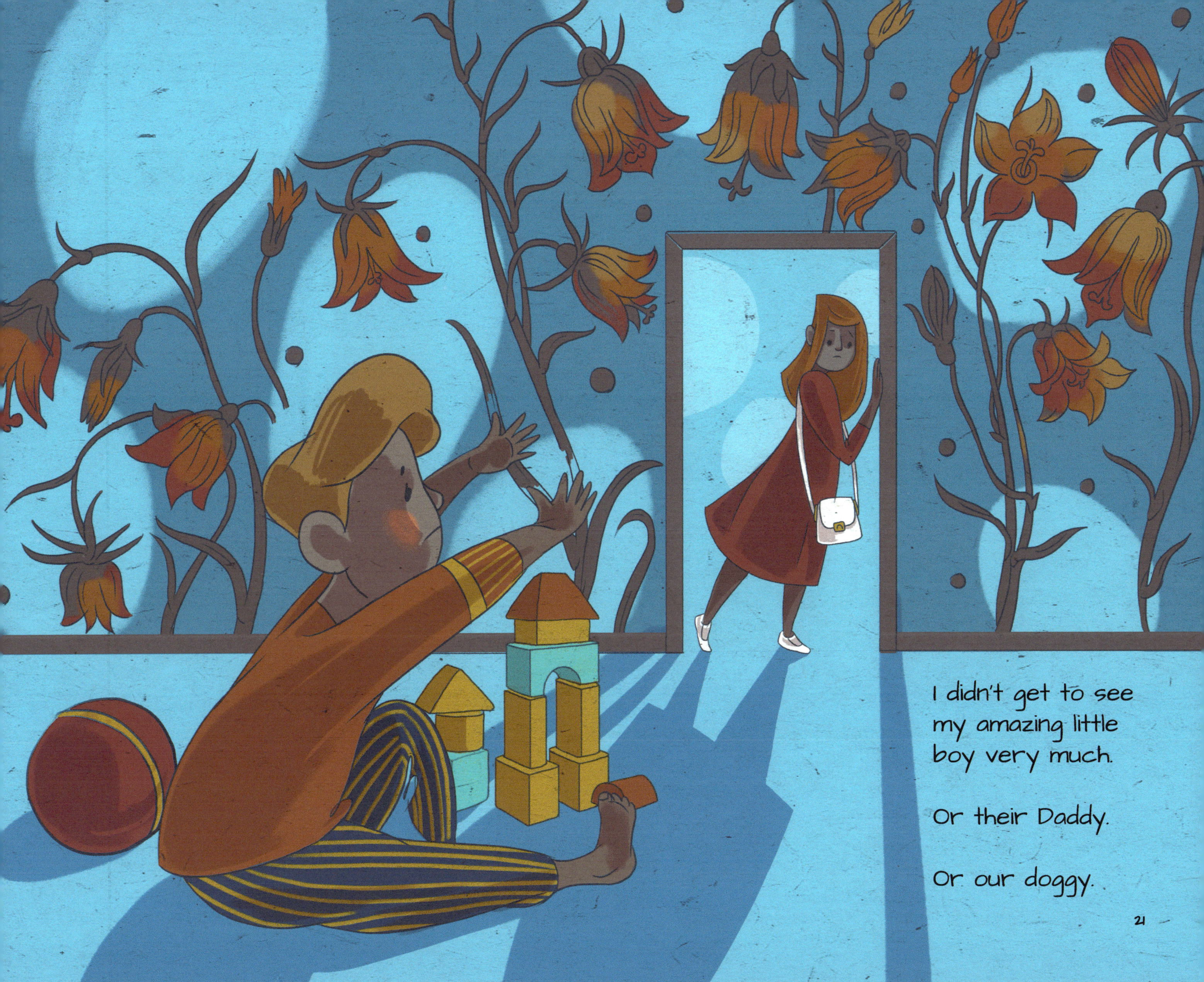

I didn't get to see
my amazing little
boy very much.

Or their Daddy.

Or our doggy.

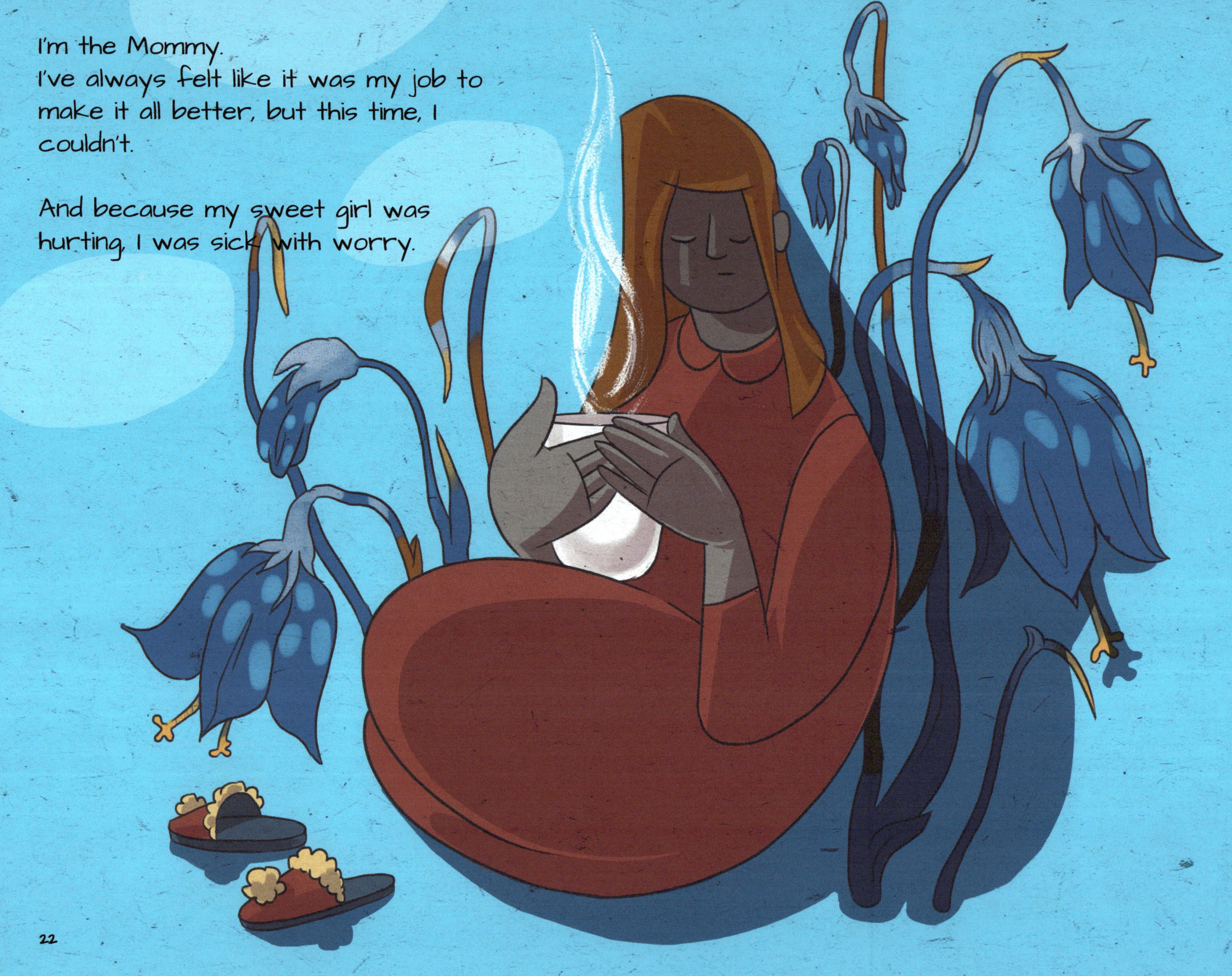

I'm the Mommy.
I've always felt like it was my job to make it all better, but this time, I couldn't.

And because my sweet girl was hurting, I was sick with worry.

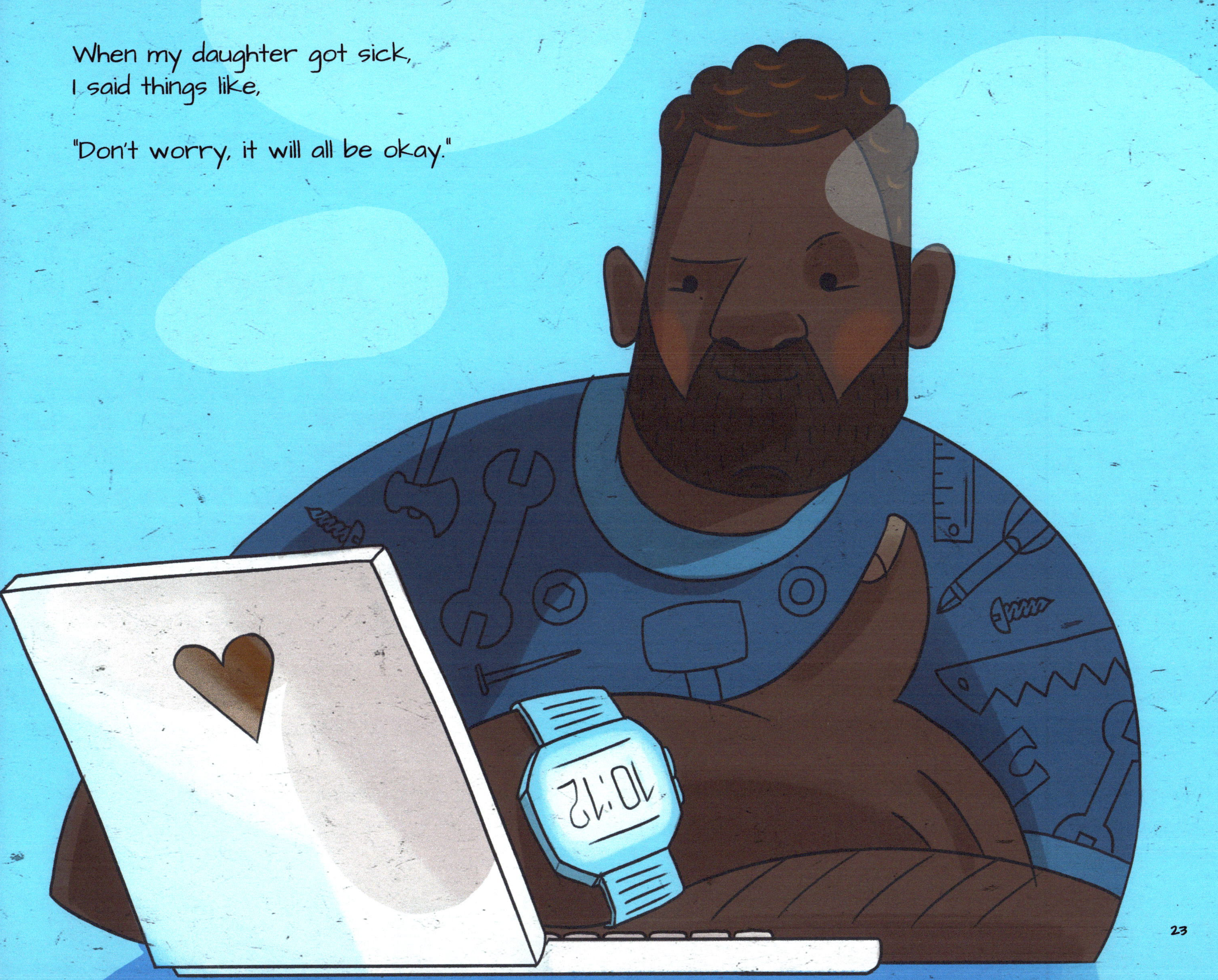

When my daughter got sick,
I said things like,

"Don't worry, it will all be okay."

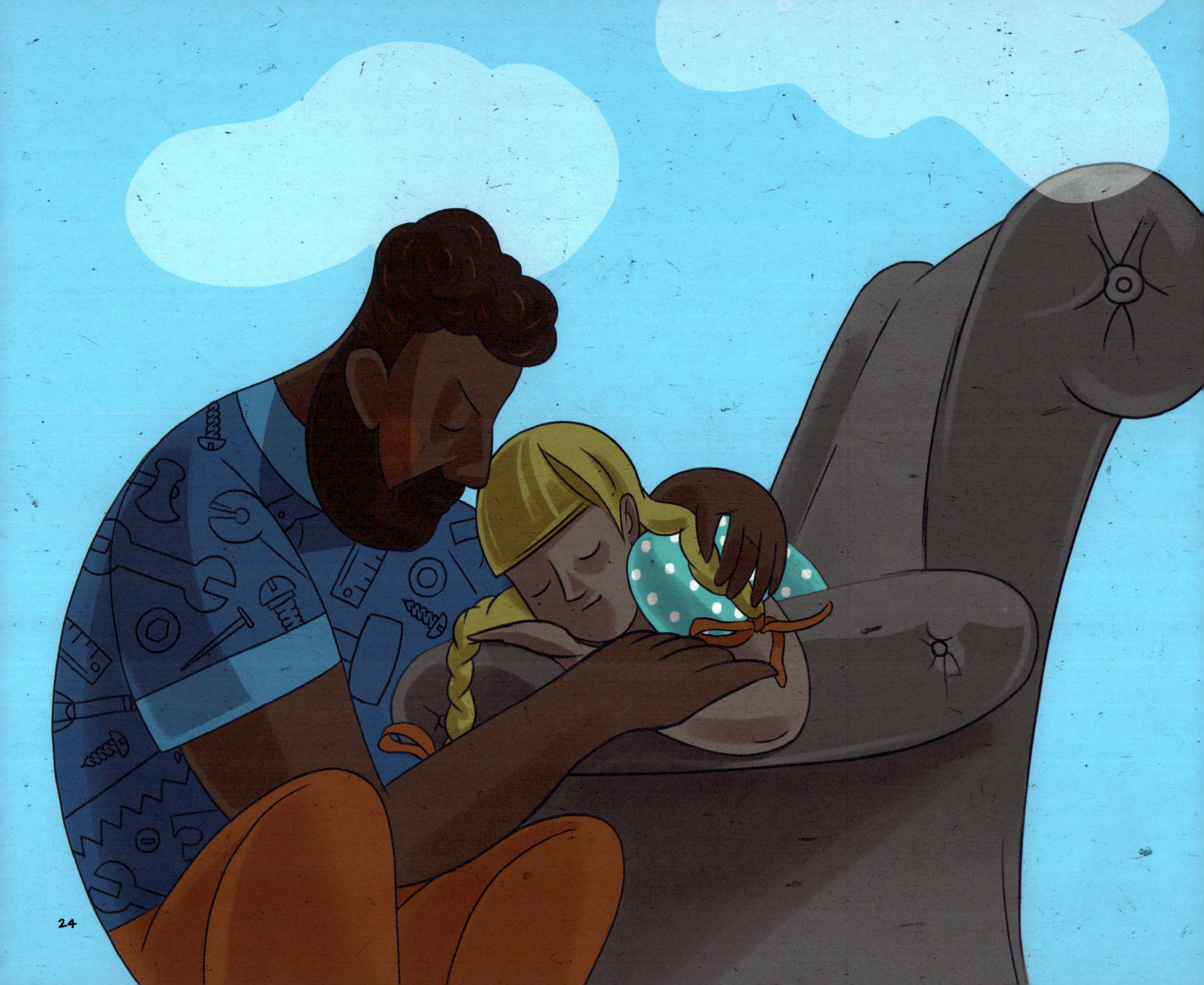

I'm the Daddy.
I've always felt like it was
my job to fix things.

I would kiss her hand or
forehead and say,
"All Better!"

But it wasn't.
I was heartsick.

When my best friend got sick,
she missed a lot of school.
And I missed her a lot.

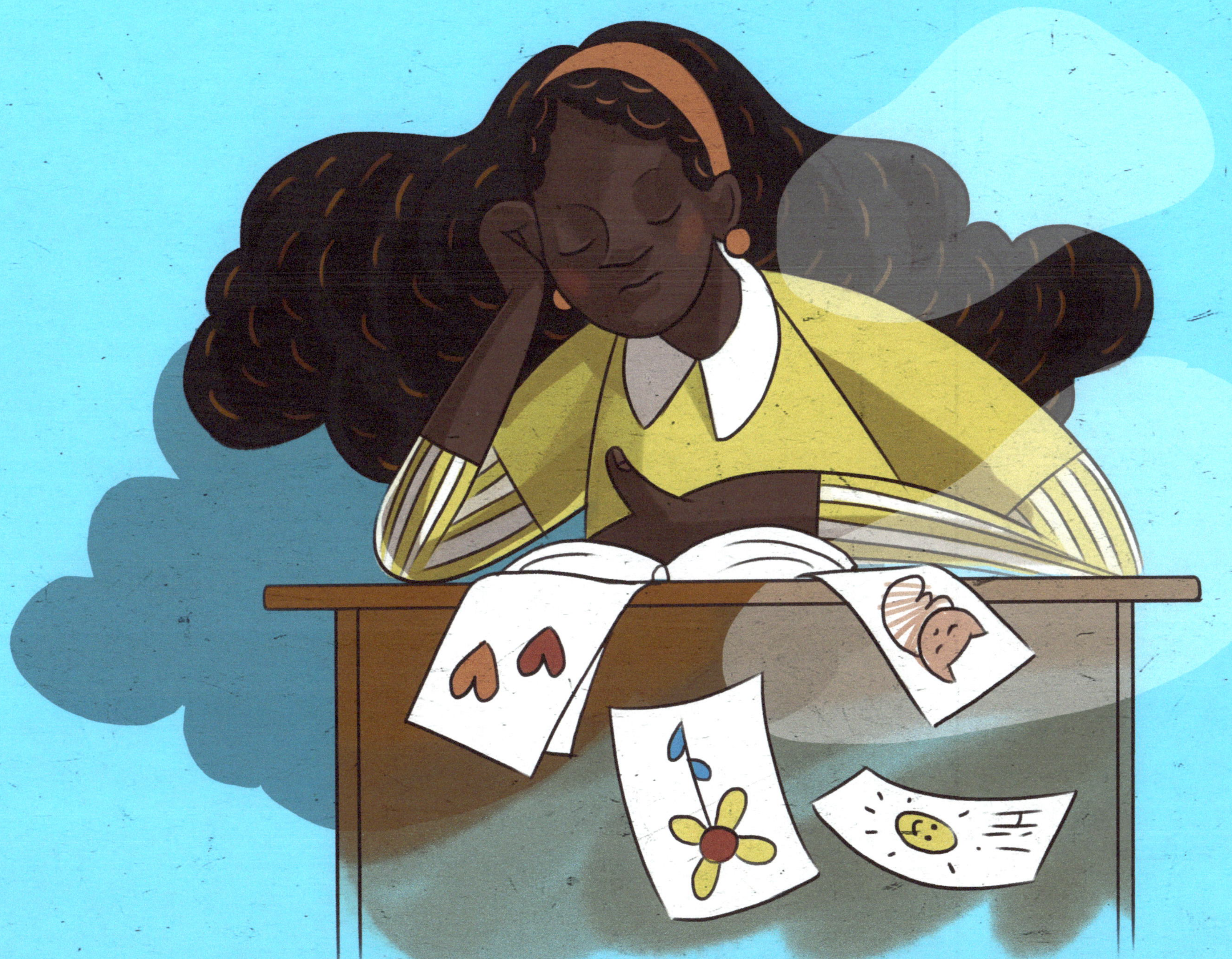

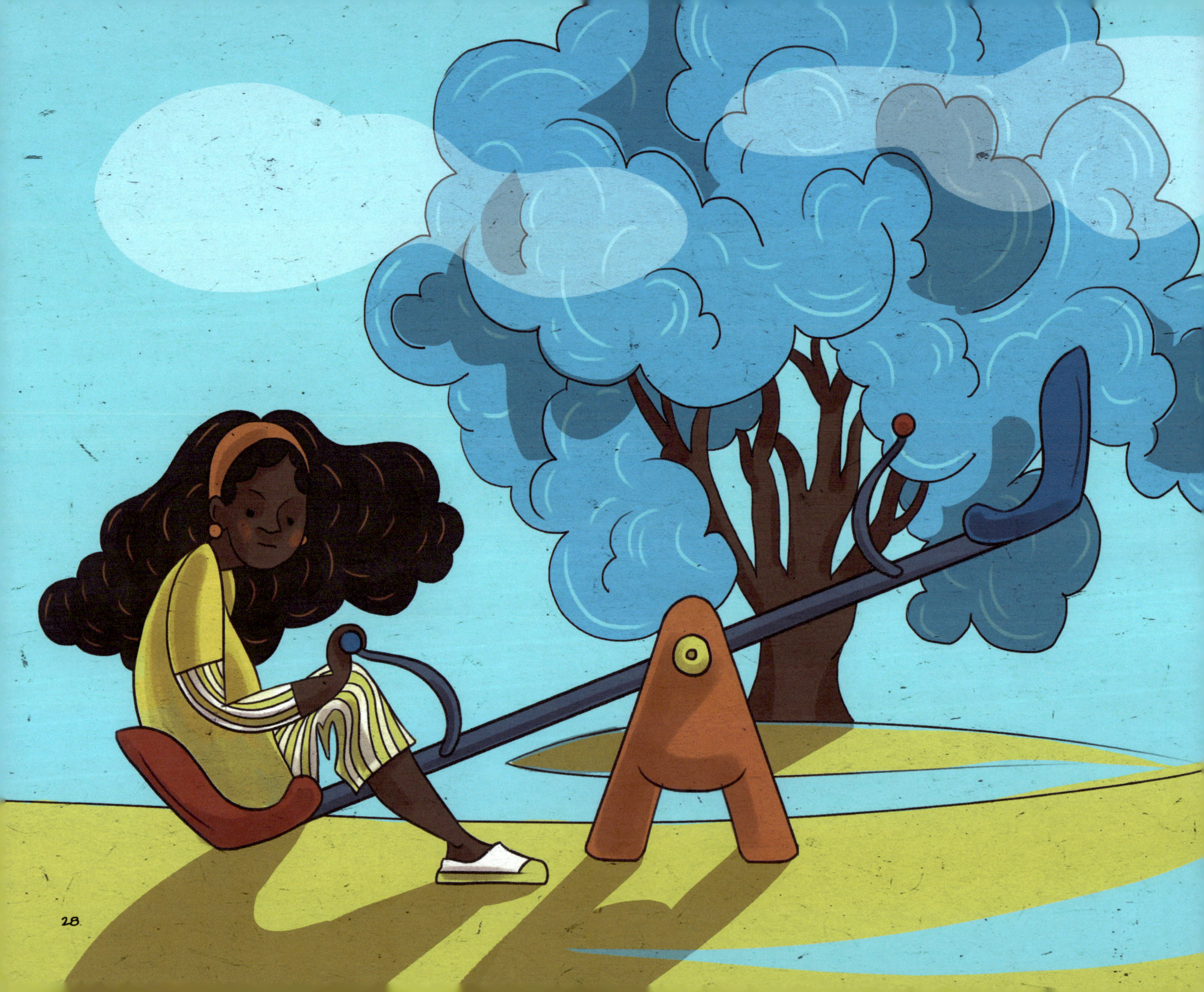

She wasn't allowed to
eat in the lunchroom with me,
be on the playground with me,
or have playdates with me.

And if I was sick,
I wasn't allowed to be with her.

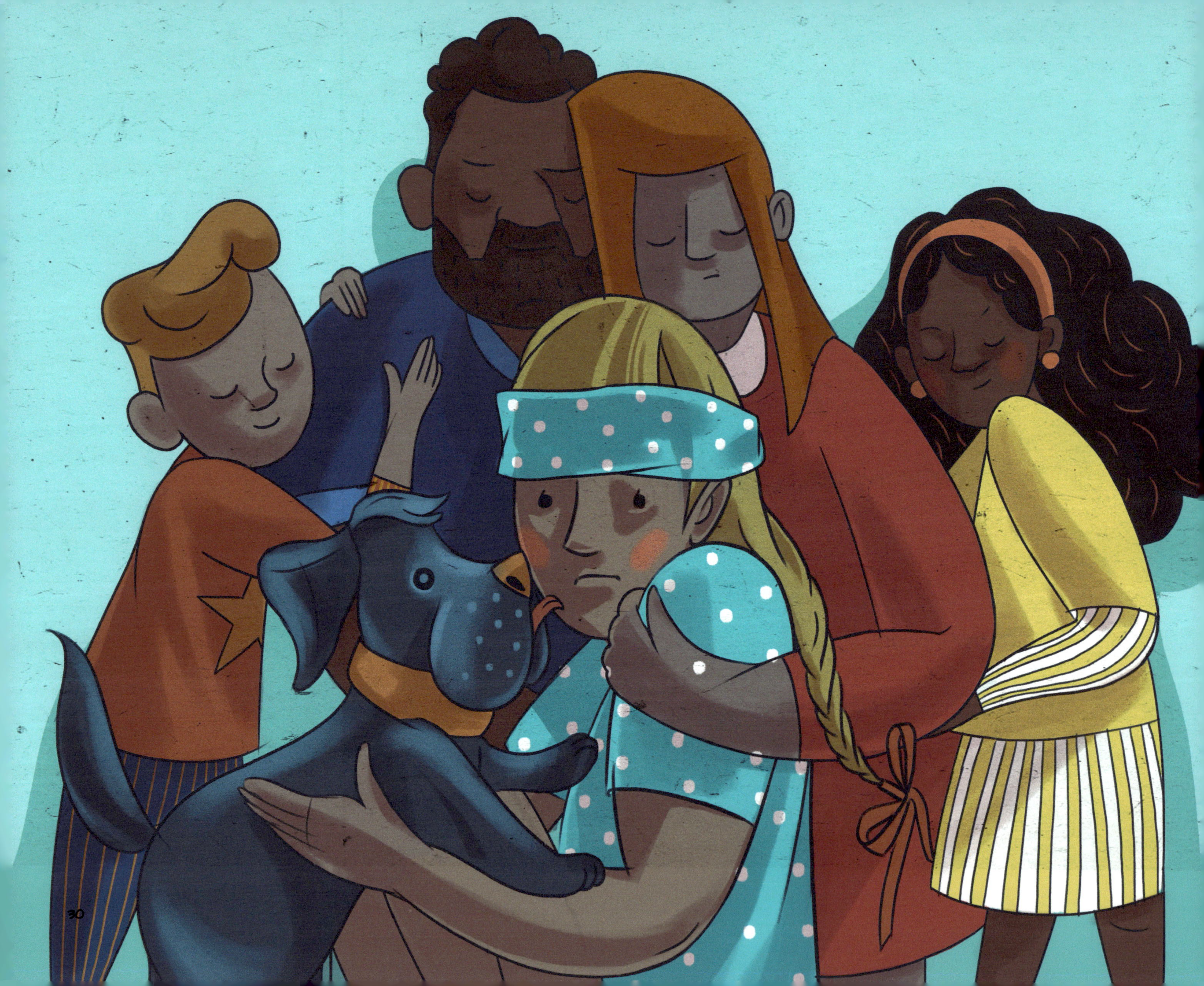

When someone you love gets sick,
it feels like everything changes.

Like, immediately.

In a way, it kind of feels like
we all get sick.

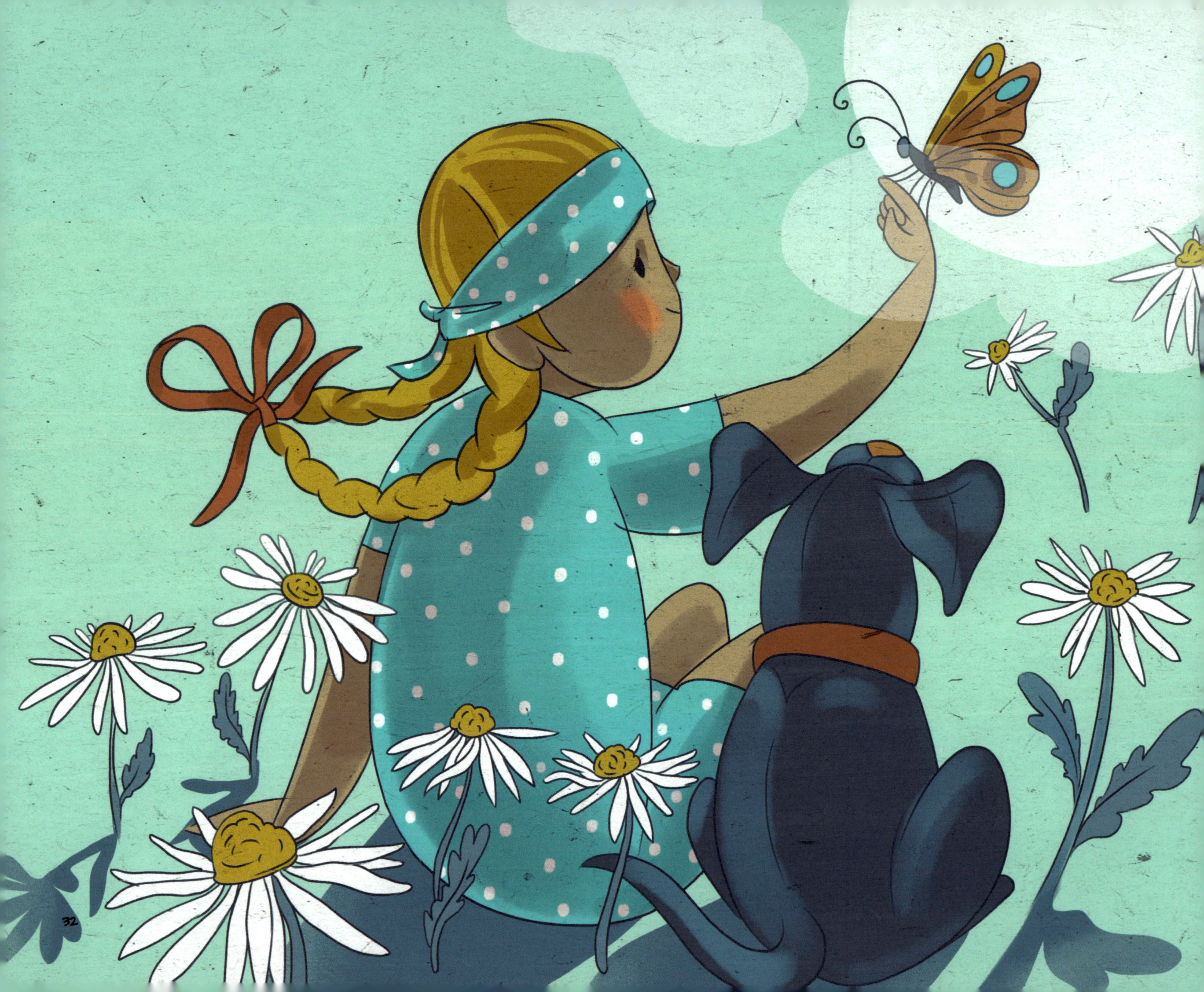

When I got sick,
it wasn't good...

But it wasn't all bad.

In fact, some unexpected nice things
also happened.

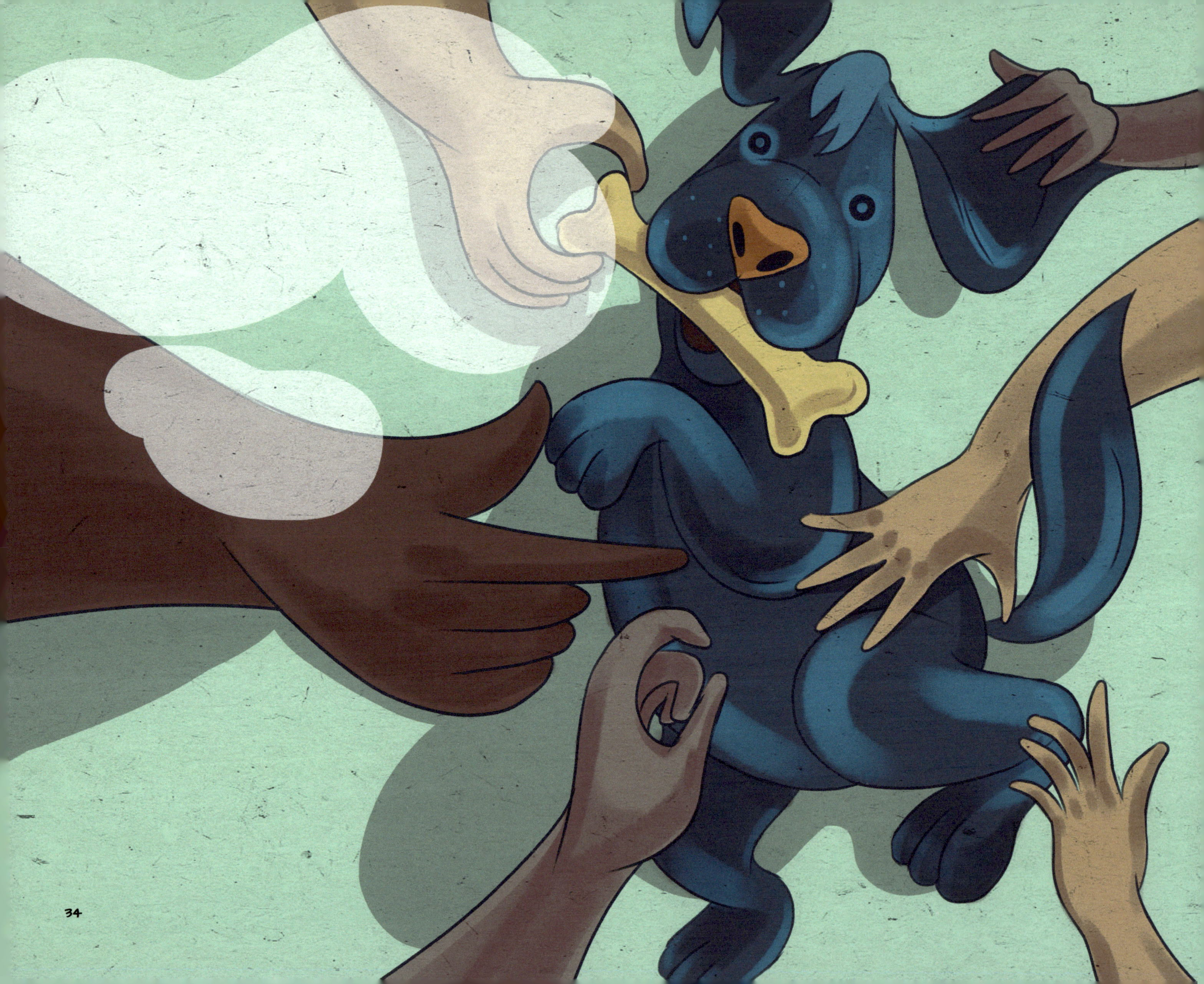

When the big girl got sick, I did get
more hugs and belly rubs.

Every one of the humans said
it made them feel better.

Which made me feel better, because
I could feel how sad they were.

(I'm still learning what not to do when
I get bored.)

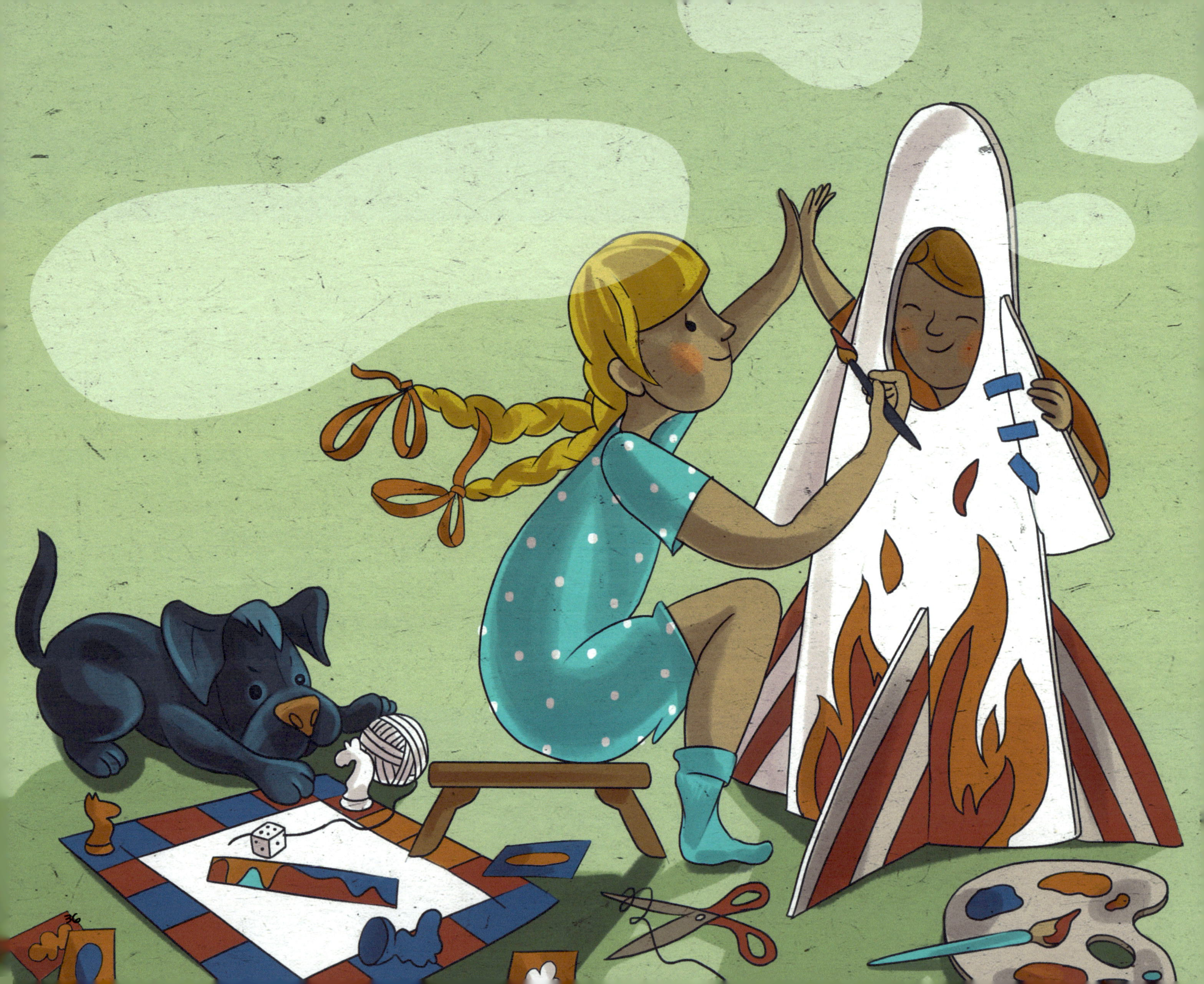

When my big sister got sick, she taught me how to play board games.
(Sometimes I even won.)

We snuggled on the sofa watching her movies.
(Don't tell anyone, but I liked them too.)

We did lots of super cool art projects together.

And on weekends, Mommy made a big stack
of my favorite pancakes and said I could eat them
all week long for breakfast, lunch and dinner if it made me happy.
It did...so I did!

Because my daughter got sick, I got a lot of
Daddy-time with my amazing son, which I will
cherish forever.

I learned a lot more about him, like
how funny he is and how truly caring he is.

And that it's okay to eat pancakes at every meal
(for a little while).

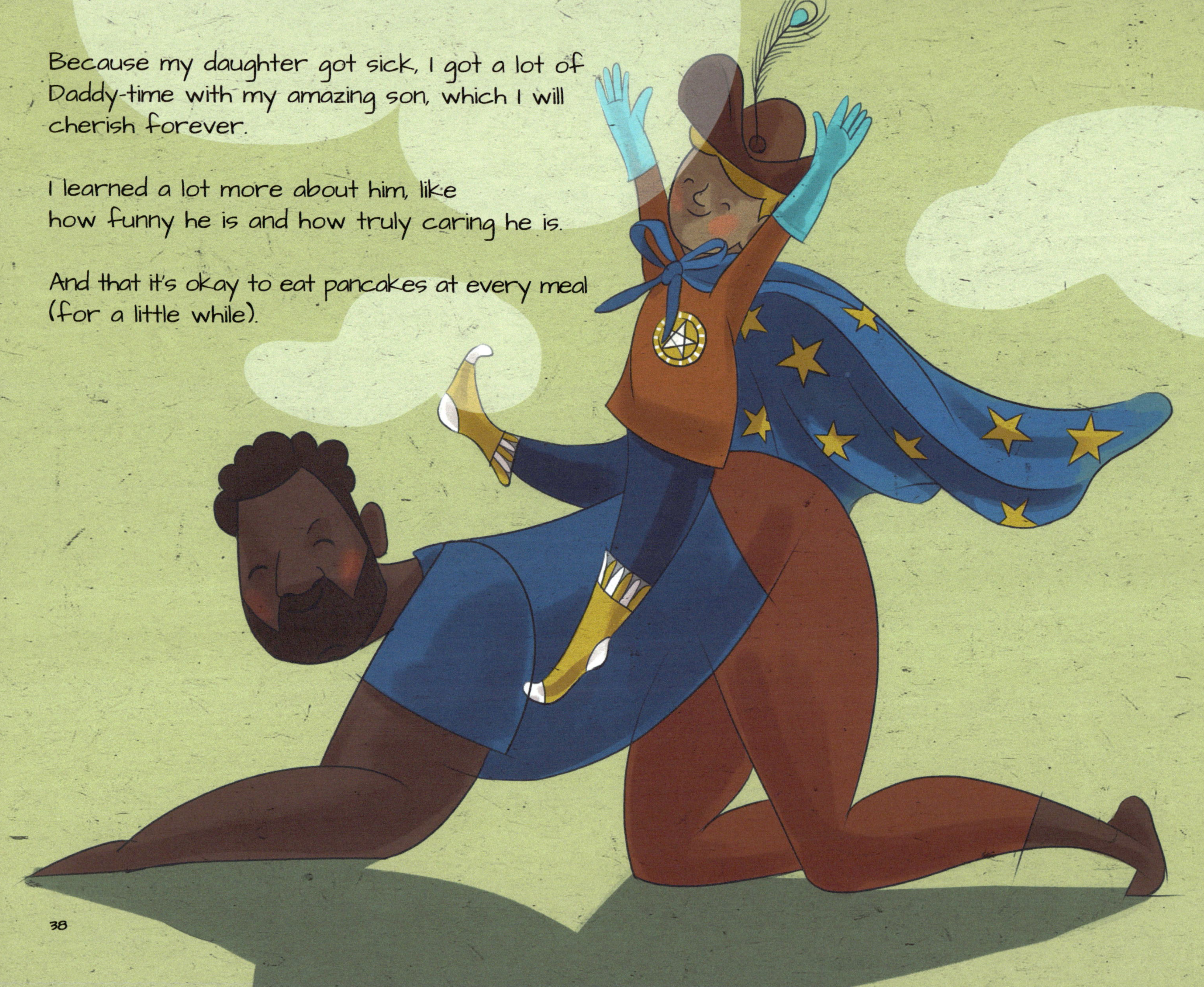

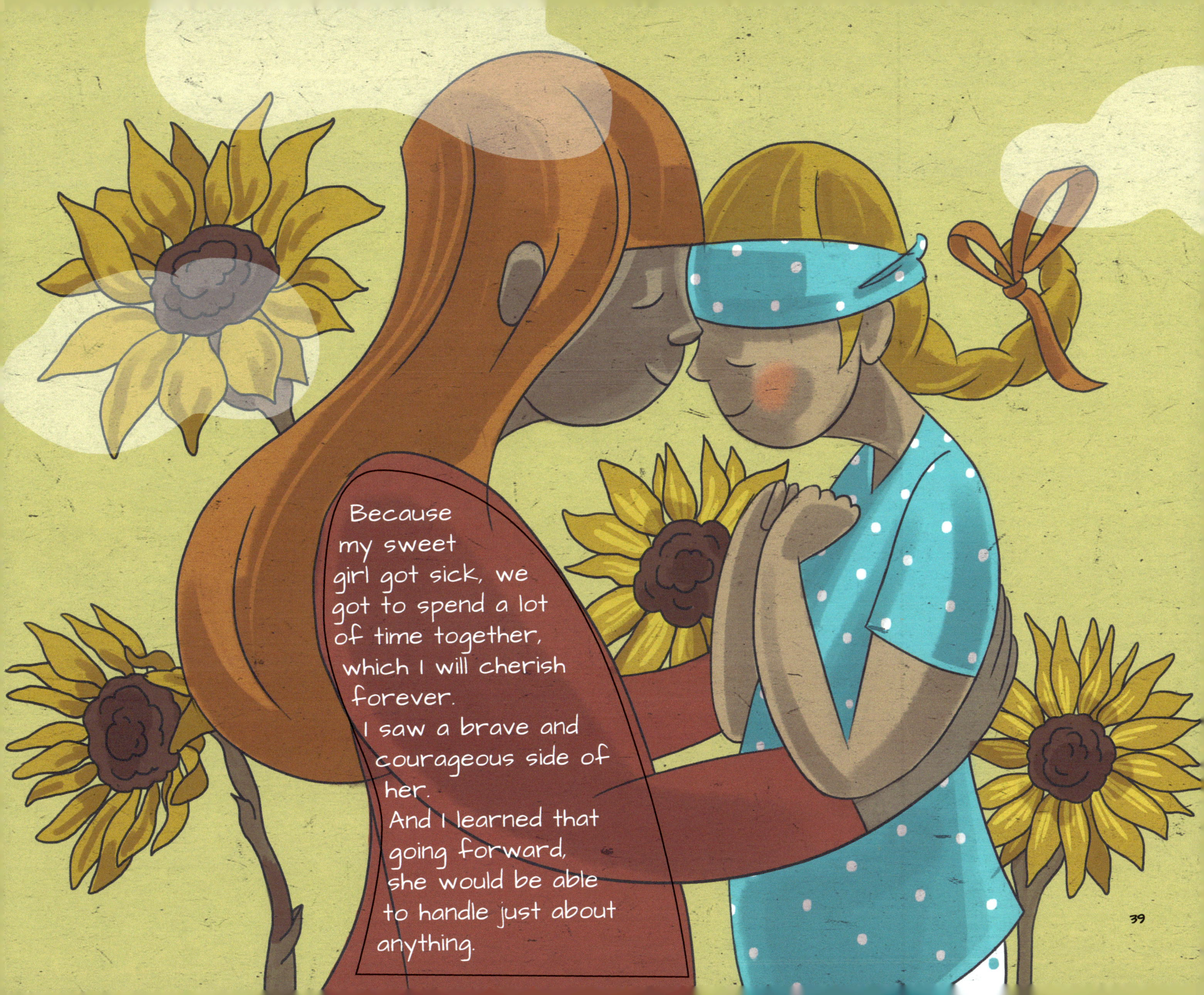

Because
my sweet
girl got sick, we
got to spend a lot
of time together,
which I will cherish
forever.
I saw a brave and
courageous side of
her.
And I learned that
going forward,
she would be able
to handle just about
anything.

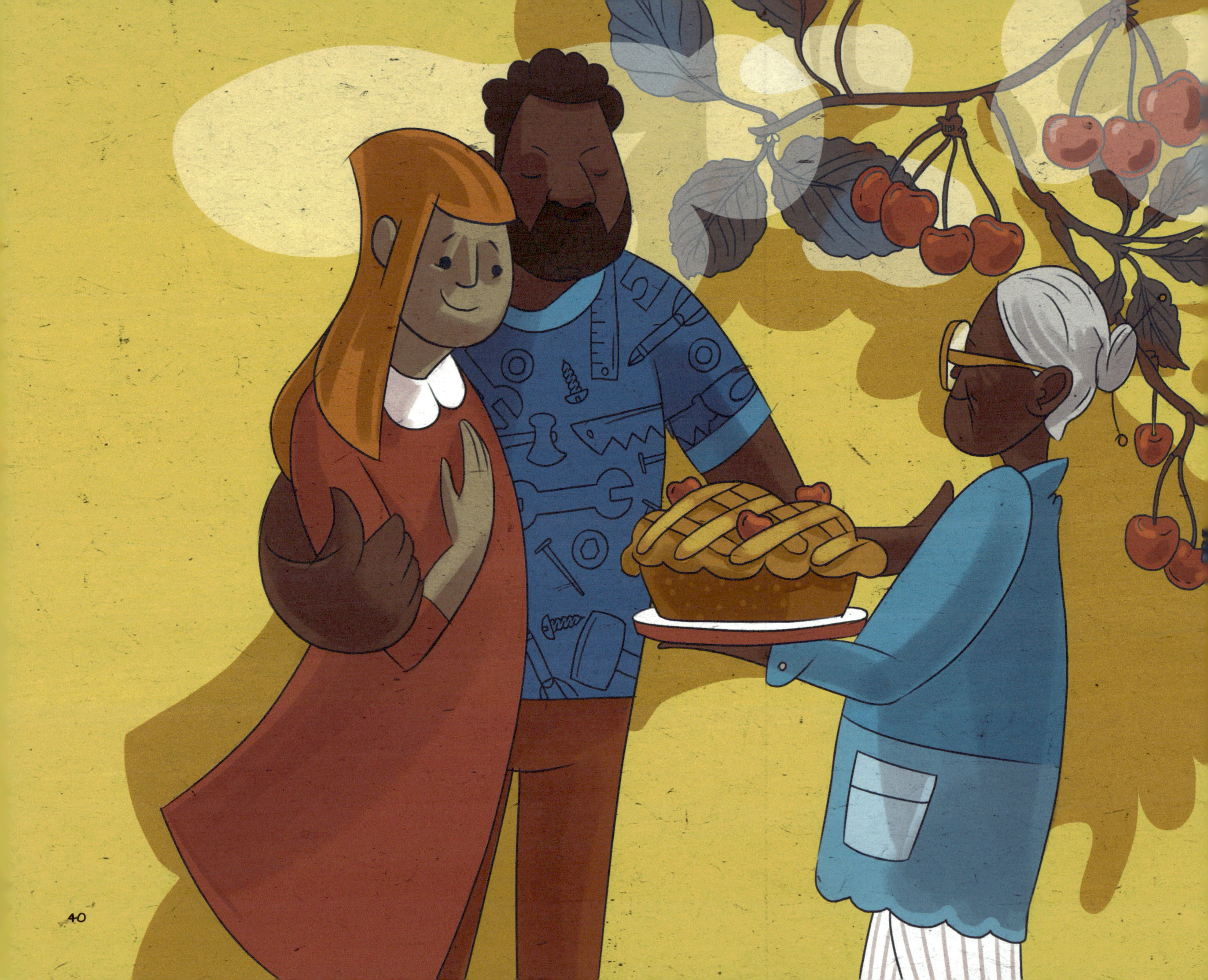

Because our sweet girl got sick,
kind and generous people
offered to help us.

And we learned it was okay to
let them.

When I got sick, I learned a Mommy's lap
is better than any pillow when you're hurting
and can't fall asleep.

I learned a Daddy can squeeze your heart
from very far away, just by saying, "I love you"
over the phone.

I learned little brothers can make it (mostly)
all better, just by sitting next to you and holding
your hand.

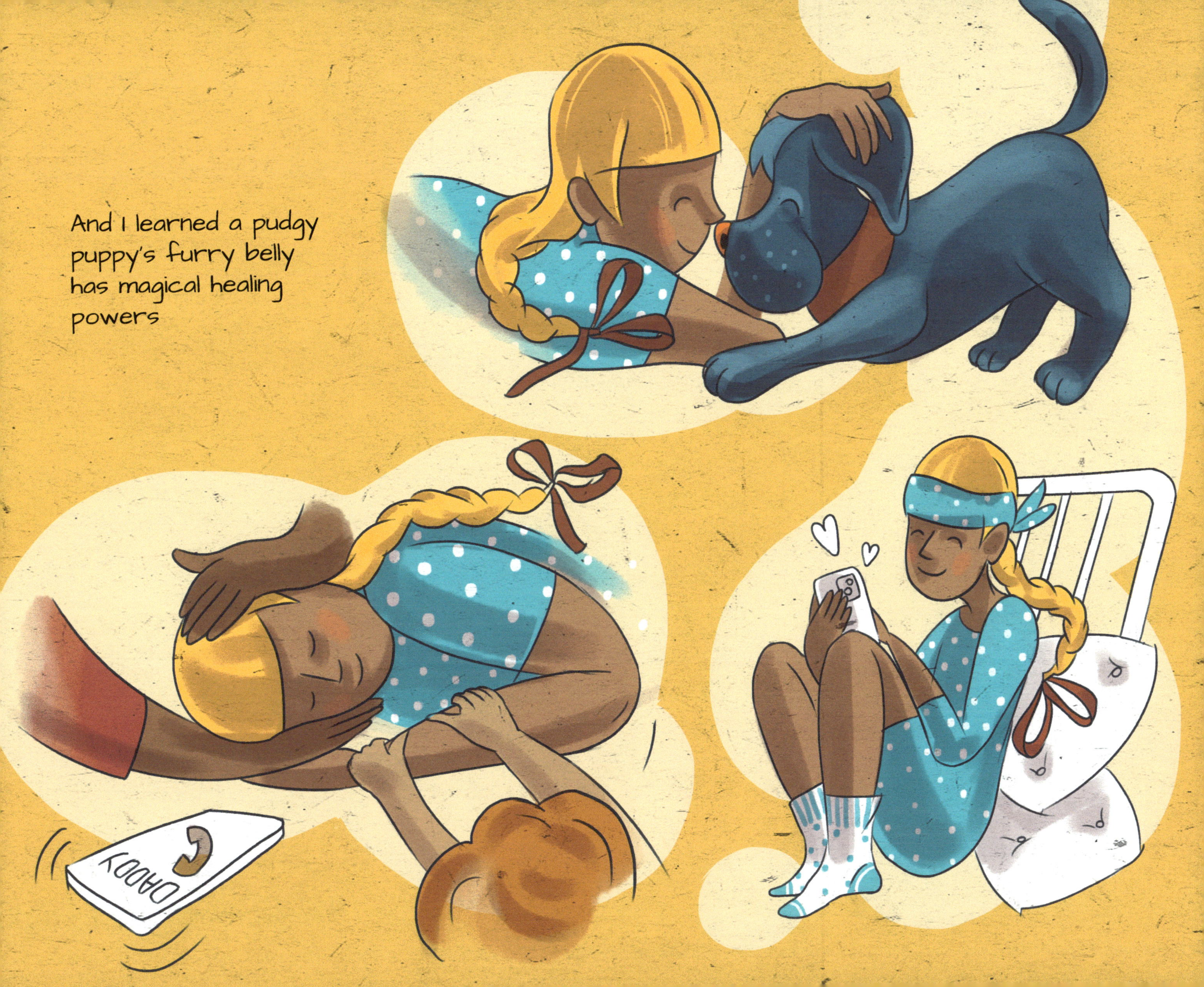
And I learned a pudgy
puppy's furry belly
has magical healing
powers
DADDY

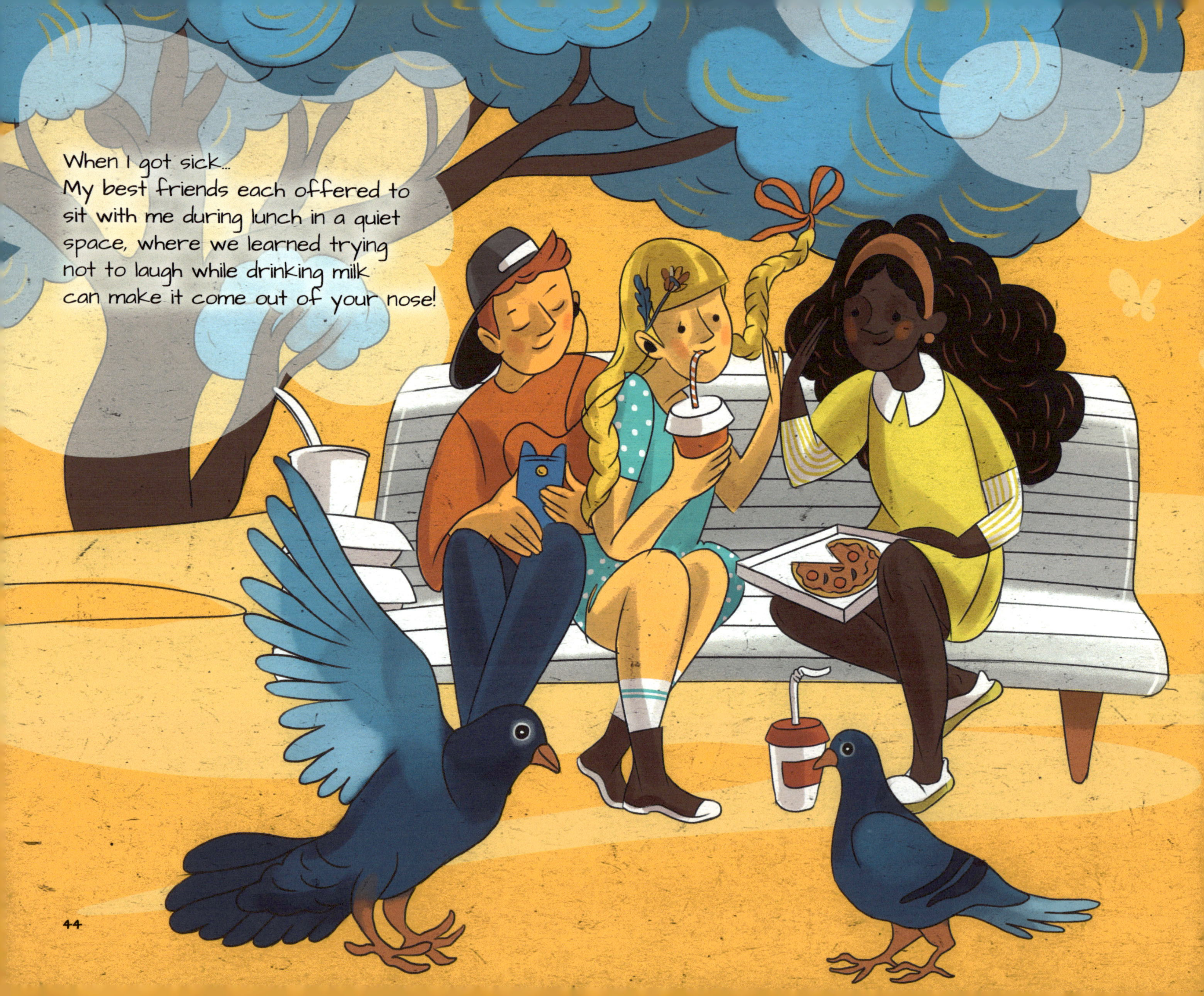

When I got sick...
My best friends each offered to
sit with me during lunch in a quiet
space, where we learned trying
not to laugh while drinking milk
can make it come out of your nose!

44

And while I was sick,
I learned something else:

It's okay to speak up for myself.
It's okay to say how I'm feeling,
especially if I'm not feeling okay.

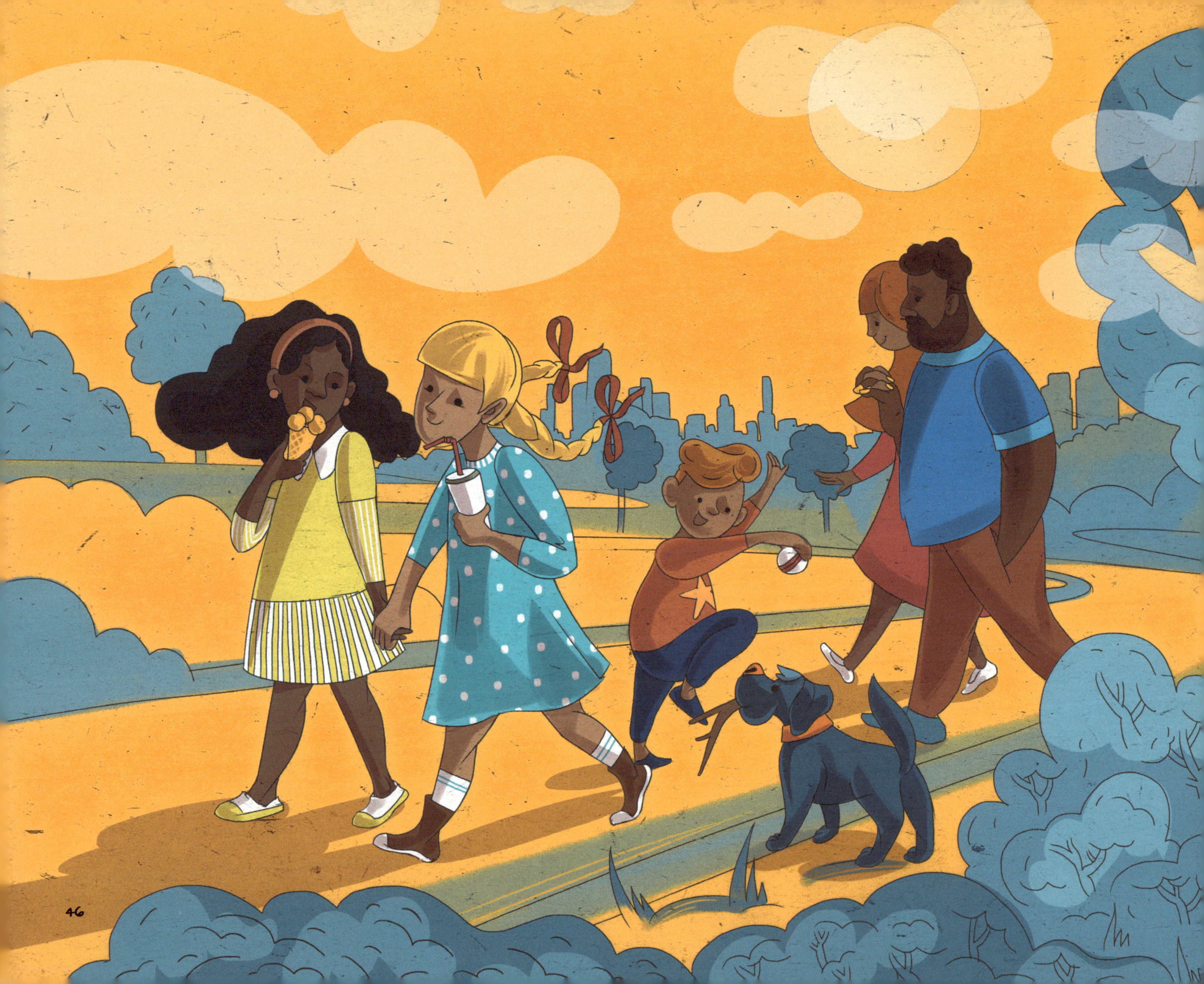

After we all got sick of being sick,
we finally found something that
made us all feel better...

Being together.

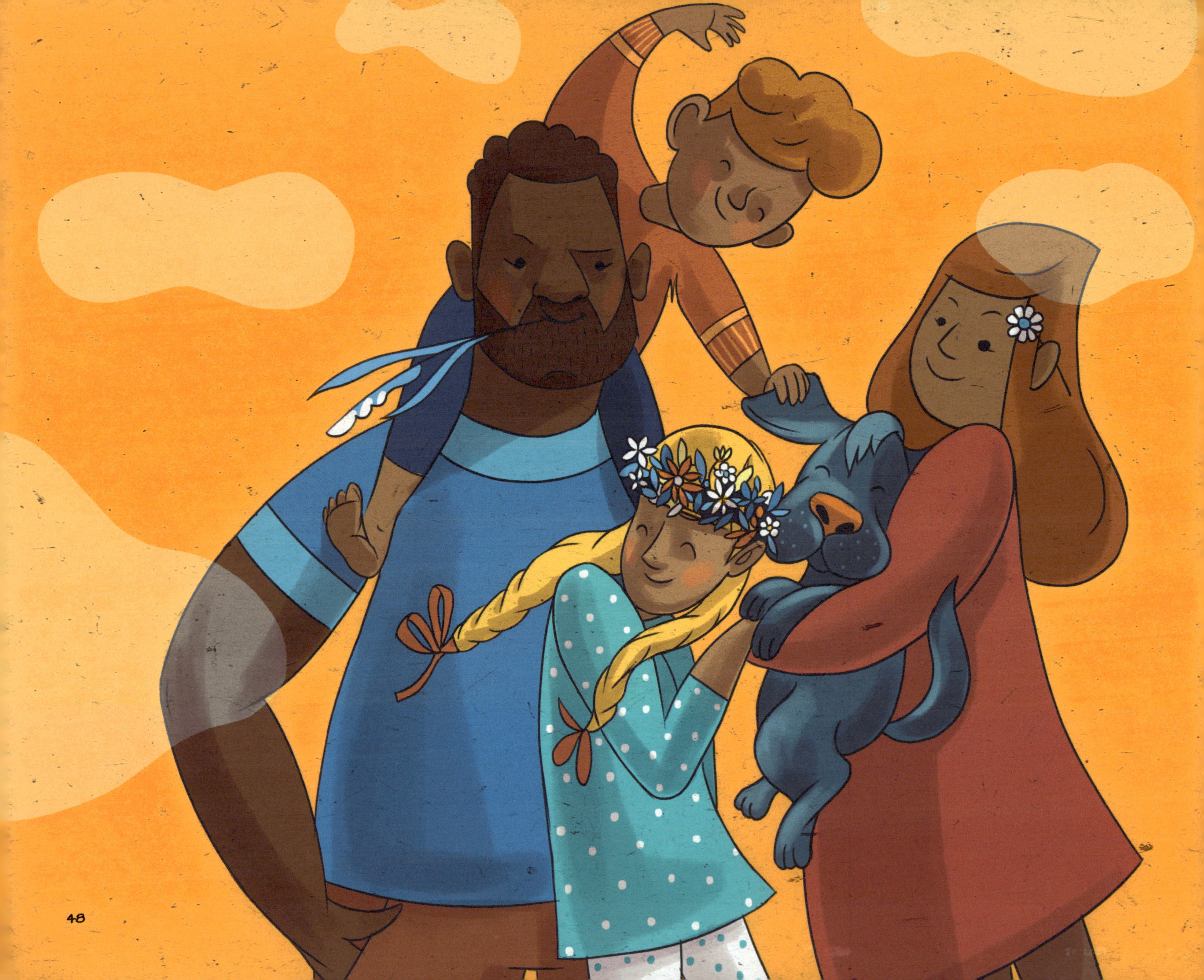

We learned to love every moment
we have together, no matter what
kind of moments they are.

Because love always lasts longer
than any day lost to being sick.

Discussion:

1. Have you or someone in your family ever been sick for a couple of days… or longer?

2. How did things change in your home?

3. How did that make you feel?

4. Did you ever feel like you wished things would just go back to normal?

5. Is there anything good you can think of that happened while you or your family member were sick?

About the Book

On October 3, 2016, 8-year-old Graysen Pendry suffered a debilitating concussion and neck injury after being hit in the head with a soccer ball. In the 3 months after the incident, she went to dozens and dozens of doctors and therapy appointments, including 3 MRI's, 2 runs to the emergency room and one very scary middle-of-the-night CAT scan. No one could figure out how to unlock her excruciating chronic headaches, neck and back pain. For 4 months, she couldn't be in class longer than 10 minutes at a time. She missed an entire year of gym class. She had to give up singing and music because the one thing that gave her so much joy now only made all the pain worse. And because the concussion threw off her balance, she fell and broke her ankle. It was a very rough 9 months before she was officially cleared of the concussion and allowed to go back to just being a kid.

During that time, Graysen's family and friends felt their lives changed, too. This is what happens when someone in your family gets sick. Everyone is asked to make changes, even a new puppy whose sole purpose in life is to make people happy. Suddenly, no one is happy. And sometimes it's really hard to sort out all the feelings that come along with changes that are forced on you.

After Graysen was cleared from her concussion, her family was so grateful she was well again, but they all realized, from a common cold or flu to very, very scary cancer, there were still a lot of people with a sick family member. They decided to share their story, so anyone else who might be feeling the same way would know they weren't alone.

About the Authors

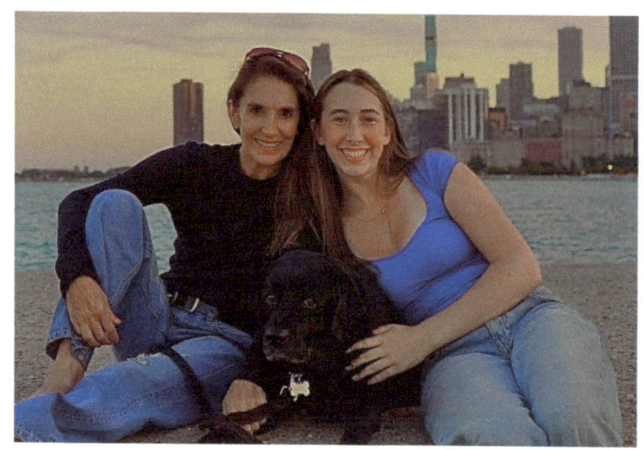

Graysen Pendry is a daughter, sister, friend, and author who has written books for young readers about her experience during the year she had her concussion.

Mac Pendry is the sweet, patient, kind, funny son, brother and friend who had lots of ideas and words for this book.

Maureen Maher is a mom, wife, daughter, friend, and storyteller.

Tom Pendry is the silently strong father, husband, brother, son and friend who would prefer to just move forward, being grateful that his family is healthy.

Paris, the English Black Labrador, is a willing participant in anything that involves belly rubs and treats-and not necessarily in that order.

About the Illustrator

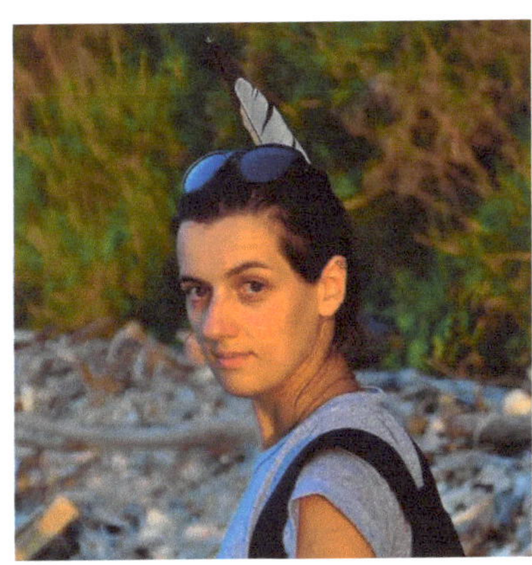

Ksenia Logovaia is a Belarusian artist and illustrator, a mom and traveller, a dog and horse lover! She comes from Minsk, Belarus and now lives in Poland. She adores drawing and painting while traveling-her sketchbook is always with her.

9 781960 876584